Blood Sugar Tr

~weekly set up to track daily
~ includes images to color for yo

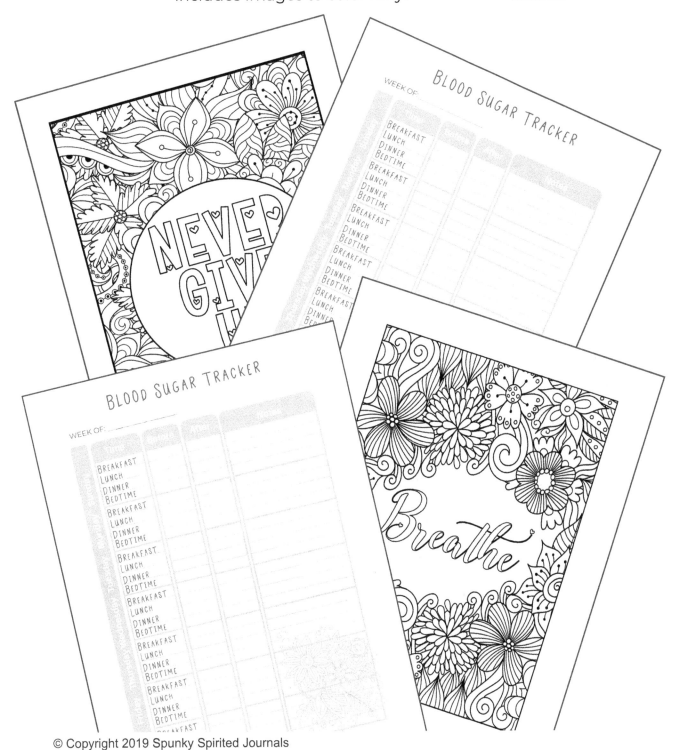

© Copyright 2019 Spunky Spirited Journals

All rights reserved.

This book or any portion thereof may not be reproduced or used in any manner whatsoever without the express written permission of the publisher except for the use of brief quotations in a book review.

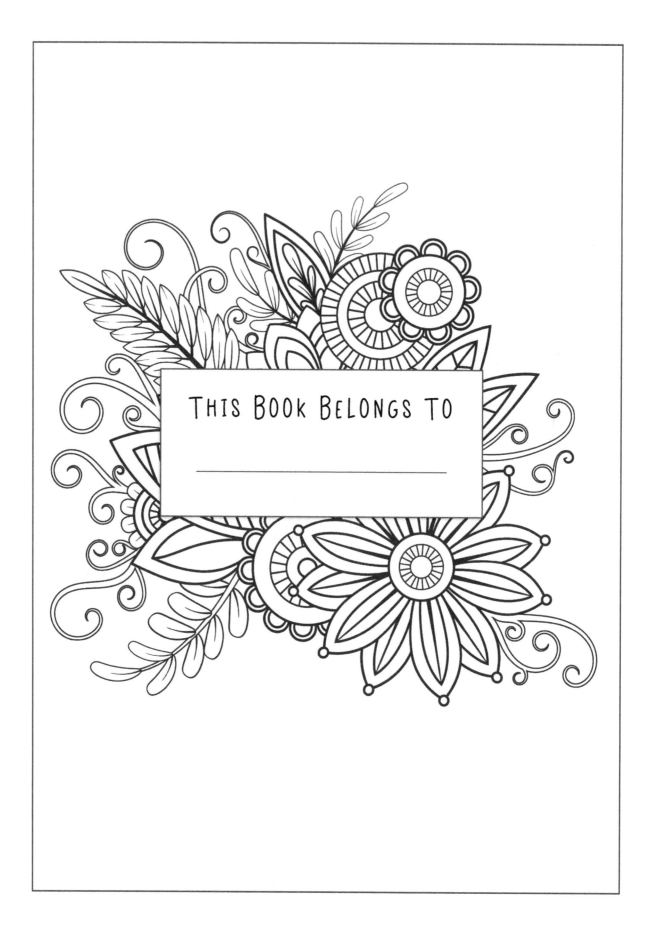

Blood Sugar Tracker

WEEK OF: _____

Day	Time	Before	After	Notes
Sunday	Breakfast			
	Lunch			
	Dinner			
	Bedtime			
Monday	Breakfast			
	Lunch			
	Dinner			
	Bedtime			
Tuesday	Breakfast			
	Lunch			
	Dinner			
	Bedtime			
Wednesday	Breakfast			
	Lunch			
	Dinner			
	Bedtime			
Thursday	Breakfast			
	Lunch			
	Dinner			
	Bedtime			
Friday	Breakfast			
	Lunch			
	Dinner			
	Bedtime			
Saturday	Breakfast			
	Lunch			
	Dinner			
	Bedtime			

Blood Sugar Tracker

WEEK OF: _____

	Time	Before	After	Notes
Sunday	Breakfast			
	Lunch			
	Dinner			
	Bedtime			
Monday	Breakfast			
	Lunch			
	Dinner			
	Bedtime			
Tuesday	Breakfast			
	Lunch			
	Dinner			
	Bedtime			
Wednesday	Breakfast			
	Lunch			
	Dinner			
	Bedtime			
Thursday	Breakfast			
	Lunch			
	Dinner			
	Bedtime			
Friday	Breakfast			
	Lunch			
	Dinner			
	Bedtime			
Saturday	Breakfast			
	Lunch			
	Dinner			
	Bedtime			

Blood Sugar Tracker

WEEK OF: _____

	Time	Before	After	Notes
Sunday	Breakfast			
	Lunch			
	Dinner			
	Bedtime			
Monday	Breakfast			
	Lunch			
	Dinner			
	Bedtime			
Tuesday	Breakfast			
	Lunch			
	Dinner			
	Bedtime			
Wednesday	Breakfast			
	Lunch			
	Dinner			
	Bedtime			
Thursday	Breakfast			
	Lunch			
	Dinner			
	Bedtime			
Friday	Breakfast			
	Lunch			
	Dinner			
	Bedtime			
Saturday	Breakfast			
	Lunch			
	Dinner			
	Bedtime			

Blood Sugar Tracker

WEEK OF: _____

	Time	Before	After	Notes
Sunday	Breakfast			
	Lunch			
	Dinner			
	Bedtime			
Monday	Breakfast			
	Lunch			
	Dinner			
	Bedtime			
Tuesday	Breakfast			
	Lunch			
	Dinner			
	Bedtime			
Wednesday	Breakfast			
	Lunch			
	Dinner			
	Bedtime			
Thursday	Breakfast			
	Lunch			
	Dinner			
	Bedtime			
Friday	Breakfast			
	Lunch			
	Dinner			
	Bedtime			
Saturday	Breakfast			
	Lunch			
	Dinner			
	Bedtime			

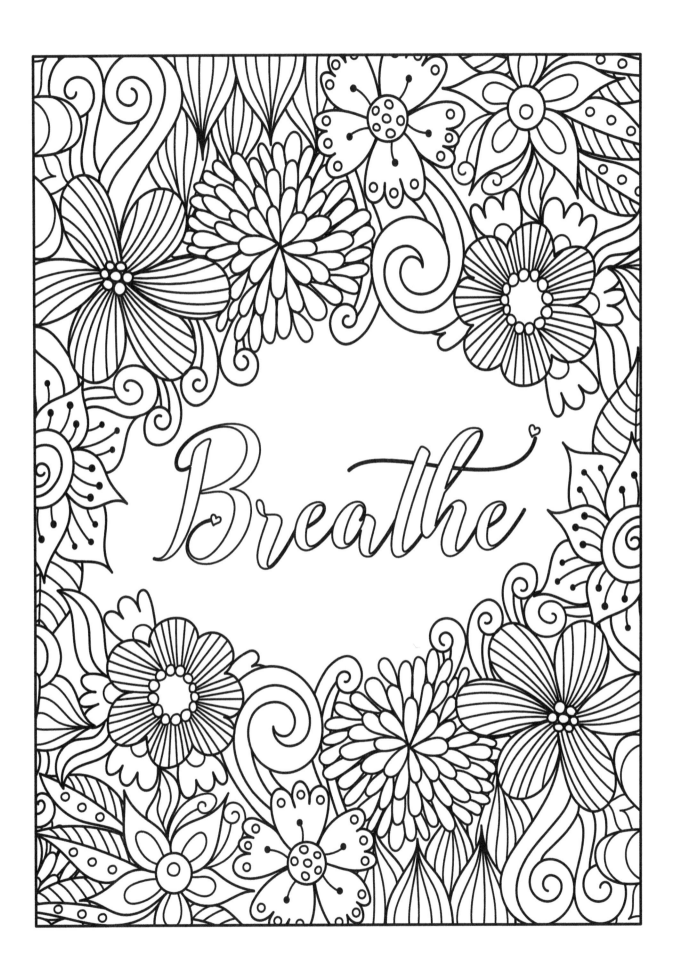

Blood Sugar Tracker

WEEK OF: _____

	Time	Before	After	Notes
Sunday	Breakfast			
	Lunch			
	Dinner			
	Bedtime			
Monday	Breakfast			
	Lunch			
	Dinner			
	Bedtime			
Tuesday	Breakfast			
	Lunch			
	Dinner			
	Bedtime			
Wednesday	Breakfast			
	Lunch			
	Dinner			
	Bedtime			
Thursday	Breakfast			
	Lunch			
	Dinner			
	Bedtime			
Friday	Breakfast			
	Lunch			
	Dinner			
	Bedtime			
Saturday	Breakfast			
	Lunch			
	Dinner			
	Bedtime			

Blood Sugar Tracker

WEEK OF: _____

	Time	Before	After	Notes
Sunday	Breakfast			
	Lunch			
	Dinner			
	Bedtime			
Monday	Breakfast			
	Lunch			
	Dinner			
	Bedtime			
Tuesday	Breakfast			
	Lunch			
	Dinner			
	Bedtime			
Wednesday	Breakfast			
	Lunch			
	Dinner			
	Bedtime			
Thursday	Breakfast			
	Lunch			
	Dinner			
	Bedtime			
Friday	Breakfast			
	Lunch			
	Dinner			
	Bedtime			
Saturday	Breakfast			
	Lunch			
	Dinner			
	Bedtime			

Blood Sugar Tracker

WEEK OF: _____

	Time	Before	After	Notes
Sunday	Breakfast			
	Lunch			
	Dinner			
	Bedtime			
Monday	Breakfast			
	Lunch			
	Dinner			
	Bedtime			
Tuesday	Breakfast			
	Lunch			
	Dinner			
	Bedtime			
Wednesday	Breakfast			
	Lunch			
	Dinner			
	Bedtime			
Thursday	Breakfast			
	Lunch			
	Dinner			
	Bedtime			
Friday	Breakfast			
	Lunch			
	Dinner			
	Bedtime			
Saturday	Breakfast			
	Lunch			
	Dinner			
	Bedtime			

Blood Sugar Tracker

WEEK OF: _____

	Time	Before	After	Notes
Sunday	Breakfast			
	Lunch			
	Dinner			
	Bedtime			
Monday	Breakfast			
	Lunch			
	Dinner			
	Bedtime			
Tuesday	Breakfast			
	Lunch			
	Dinner			
	Bedtime			
Wednesday	Breakfast			
	Lunch			
	Dinner			
	Bedtime			
Thursday	Breakfast			
	Lunch			
	Dinner			
	Bedtime			
Friday	Breakfast			
	Lunch			
	Dinner			
	Bedtime			
Saturday	Breakfast			
	Lunch			
	Dinner			
	Bedtime			

NOTES:

Blood Sugar Tracker

WEEK OF: _____

	Time	Before	After	Notes
Sunday	Breakfast Lunch Dinner Bedtime			
Monday	Breakfast Lunch Dinner Bedtime			
Tuesday	Breakfast Lunch Dinner Bedtime			
Wednesday	Breakfast Lunch Dinner Bedtime			
Thursday	Breakfast Lunch Dinner Bedtime			
Friday	Breakfast Lunch Dinner Bedtime			
Saturday	Breakfast Lunch Dinner Bedtime			

Blood Sugar Tracker

WEEK OF: _____

	Time	Before	After	Notes
Sunday	Breakfast			
	Lunch			
	Dinner			
	Bedtime			
Monday	Breakfast			
	Lunch			
	Dinner			
	Bedtime			
Tuesday	Breakfast			
	Lunch			
	Dinner			
	Bedtime			
Wednesday	Breakfast			
	Lunch			
	Dinner			
	Bedtime			
Thursday	Breakfast			
	Lunch			
	Dinner			
	Bedtime			
Friday	Breakfast			
	Lunch			
	Dinner			
	Bedtime			
Saturday	Breakfast			
	Lunch			
	Dinner			
	Bedtime			

Blood Sugar Tracker

WEEK OF: _____

Day	Time	Before	After	Notes
Sunday	Breakfast			
	Lunch			
	Dinner			
	Bedtime			
Monday	Breakfast			
	Lunch			
	Dinner			
	Bedtime			
Tuesday	Breakfast			
	Lunch			
	Dinner			
	Bedtime			
Wednesday	Breakfast			
	Lunch			
	Dinner			
	Bedtime			
Thursday	Breakfast			
	Lunch			
	Dinner			
	Bedtime			
Friday	Breakfast			
	Lunch			
	Dinner			
	Bedtime			
Saturday	Breakfast			
	Lunch			
	Dinner			
	Bedtime			

Blood Sugar Tracker

WEEK OF: _____

	Time	Before	After	Notes
Sunday	Breakfast			
	Lunch			
	Dinner			
	Bedtime			
Monday	Breakfast			
	Lunch			
	Dinner			
	Bedtime			
Tuesday	Breakfast			
	Lunch			
	Dinner			
	Bedtime			
Wednesday	Breakfast			
	Lunch			
	Dinner			
	Bedtime			
Thursday	Breakfast			
	Lunch			
	Dinner			
	Bedtime			
Friday	Breakfast			
	Lunch			
	Dinner			
	Bedtime			
Saturday	Breakfast			
	Lunch			
	Dinner			
	Bedtime			

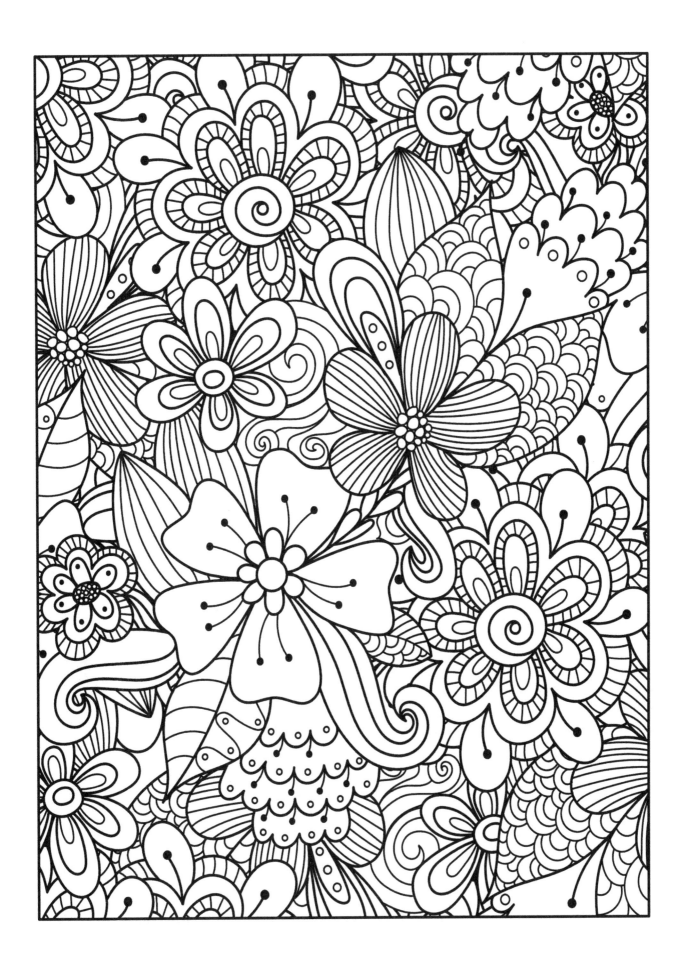

Blood Sugar Tracker

WEEK OF: _____

Day	Time	Before	After	Notes
Sunday	Breakfast			
	Lunch			
	Dinner			
	Bedtime			
Monday	Breakfast			
	Lunch			
	Dinner			
	Bedtime			
Tuesday	Breakfast			
	Lunch			
	Dinner			
	Bedtime			
Wednesday	Breakfast			
	Lunch			
	Dinner			
	Bedtime			
Thursday	Breakfast			
	Lunch			
	Dinner			
	Bedtime			
Friday	Breakfast			
	Lunch			
	Dinner			
	Bedtime			
Saturday	Breakfast			
	Lunch			
	Dinner			
	Bedtime			

Blood Sugar Tracker

WEEK OF: _____

Day	Time	Before	After	Notes
Sunday	Breakfast			
	Lunch			
	Dinner			
	Bedtime			
Monday	Breakfast			
	Lunch			
	Dinner			
	Bedtime			
Tuesday	Breakfast			
	Lunch			
	Dinner			
	Bedtime			
Wednesday	Breakfast			
	Lunch			
	Dinner			
	Bedtime			
Thursday	Breakfast			
	Lunch			
	Dinner			
	Bedtime			
Friday	Breakfast			
	Lunch			
	Dinner			
	Bedtime			
Saturday	Breakfast			
	Lunch			
	Dinner			
	Bedtime			

Blood Sugar Tracker

WEEK OF: _____

	Time	Before	After	Notes
Sunday	Breakfast			
	Lunch			
	Dinner			
	Bedtime			
Monday	Breakfast			
	Lunch			
	Dinner			
	Bedtime			
Tuesday	Breakfast			
	Lunch			
	Dinner			
	Bedtime			
Wednesday	Breakfast			
	Lunch			
	Dinner			
	Bedtime			
Thursday	Breakfast			
	Lunch			
	Dinner			
	Bedtime			
Friday	Breakfast			
	Lunch			
	Dinner			
	Bedtime			
Saturday	Breakfast			
	Lunch			
	Dinner			
	Bedtime			

Blood Sugar Tracker

WEEK OF: _____

Day	Time	Before	After	Notes
Sunday	Breakfast			
	Lunch			
	Dinner			
	Bedtime			
Monday	Breakfast			
	Lunch			
	Dinner			
	Bedtime			
Tuesday	Breakfast			
	Lunch			
	Dinner			
	Bedtime			
Wednesday	Breakfast			
	Lunch			
	Dinner			
	Bedtime			
Thursday	Breakfast			
	Lunch			
	Dinner			
	Bedtime			
Friday	Breakfast			
	Lunch			
	Dinner			
	Bedtime			
Saturday	Breakfast			
	Lunch			
	Dinner			
	Bedtime			

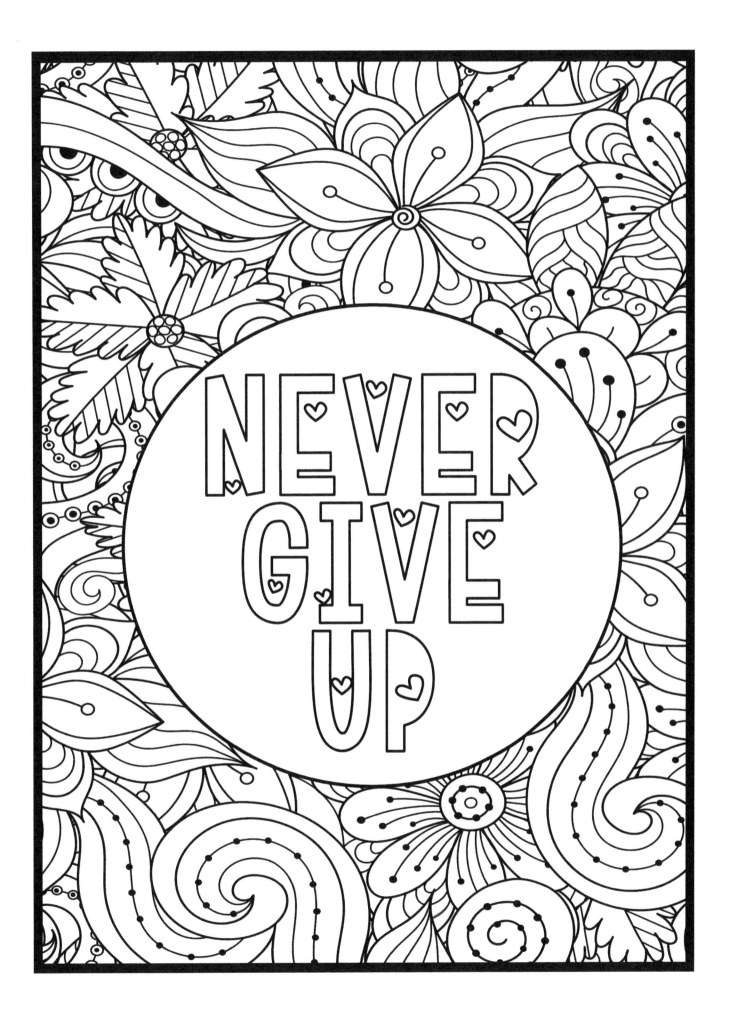

Blood Sugar Tracker

WEEK OF: _____

	Time	Before	After	Notes
Sunday	Breakfast			
	Lunch			
	Dinner			
	Bedtime			
Monday	Breakfast			
	Lunch			
	Dinner			
	Bedtime			
Tuesday	Breakfast			
	Lunch			
	Dinner			
	Bedtime			
Wednesday	Breakfast			
	Lunch			
	Dinner			
	Bedtime			
Thursday	Breakfast			
	Lunch			
	Dinner			
	Bedtime			
Friday	Breakfast			
	Lunch			
	Dinner			
	Bedtime			
Saturday	Breakfast			
	Lunch			
	Dinner			
	Bedtime			

Blood Sugar Tracker

WEEK OF: _____

Day	Time	Before	After	Notes
Sunday	Breakfast			
	Lunch			
	Dinner			
	Bedtime			
Monday	Breakfast			
	Lunch			
	Dinner			
	Bedtime			
Tuesday	Breakfast			
	Lunch			
	Dinner			
	Bedtime			
Wednesday	Breakfast			
	Lunch			
	Dinner			
	Bedtime			
Thursday	Breakfast			
	Lunch			
	Dinner			
	Bedtime			
Friday	Breakfast			
	Lunch			
	Dinner			
	Bedtime			
Saturday	Breakfast			
	Lunch			
	Dinner			
	Bedtime			

Blood Sugar Tracker

WEEK OF: _____

	Time	Before	After	Notes
Sunday	Breakfast			
	Lunch			
	Dinner			
	Bedtime			
Monday	Breakfast			
	Lunch			
	Dinner			
	Bedtime			
Tuesday	Breakfast			
	Lunch			
	Dinner			
	Bedtime			
Wednesday	Breakfast			
	Lunch			
	Dinner			
	Bedtime			
Thursday	Breakfast			
	Lunch			
	Dinner			
	Bedtime			
Friday	Breakfast			
	Lunch			
	Dinner			
	Bedtime			
Saturday	Breakfast			
	Lunch			
	Dinner			
	Bedtime			

Blood Sugar Tracker

WEEK OF: _____

	Time	Before	After	Notes
Sunday	Breakfast			
	Lunch			
	Dinner			
	Bedtime			
Monday	Breakfast			
	Lunch			
	Dinner			
	Bedtime			
Tuesday	Breakfast			
	Lunch			
	Dinner			
	Bedtime			
Wednesday	Breakfast			
	Lunch			
	Dinner			
	Bedtime			
Thursday	Breakfast			
	Lunch			
	Dinner			
	Bedtime			
Friday	Breakfast			
	Lunch			
	Dinner			
	Bedtime			
Saturday	Breakfast			
	Lunch			
	Dinner			
	Bedtime			

Blood Sugar Tracker

WEEK OF: _____

	Time	Before	After	Notes
Sunday	Breakfast			
	Lunch			
	Dinner			
	Bedtime			
Monday	Breakfast			
	Lunch			
	Dinner			
	Bedtime			
Tuesday	Breakfast			
	Lunch			
	Dinner			
	Bedtime			
Wednesday	Breakfast			
	Lunch			
	Dinner			
	Bedtime			
Thursday	Breakfast			
	Lunch			
	Dinner			
	Bedtime			
Friday	Breakfast			
	Lunch			
	Dinner			
	Bedtime			
Saturday	Breakfast			
	Lunch			
	Dinner			
	Bedtime			

Blood Sugar Tracker

WEEK OF: _____

Day	Time	Before	After	Notes
Sunday	Breakfast			
	Lunch			
	Dinner			
	Bedtime			
Monday	Breakfast			
	Lunch			
	Dinner			
	Bedtime			
Tuesday	Breakfast			
	Lunch			
	Dinner			
	Bedtime			
Wednesday	Breakfast			
	Lunch			
	Dinner			
	Bedtime			
Thursday	Breakfast			
	Lunch			
	Dinner			
	Bedtime			
Friday	Breakfast			
	Lunch			
	Dinner			
	Bedtime			
Saturday	Breakfast			
	Lunch			
	Dinner			
	Bedtime			

Blood Sugar Tracker

WEEK OF: _____

	Time	Before	After	Notes
Sunday	Breakfast			
	Lunch			
	Dinner			
	Bedtime			
Monday	Breakfast			
	Lunch			
	Dinner			
	Bedtime			
Tuesday	Breakfast			
	Lunch			
	Dinner			
	Bedtime			
Wednesday	Breakfast			
	Lunch			
	Dinner			
	Bedtime			
Thursday	Breakfast			
	Lunch			
	Dinner			
	Bedtime			
Friday	Breakfast			
	Lunch			
	Dinner			
	Bedtime			
Saturday	Breakfast			
	Lunch			
	Dinner			
	Bedtime			

Blood Sugar Tracker

WEEK OF: _____

	Time	Before	After	Notes
Sunday	Breakfast			
	Lunch			
	Dinner			
	Bedtime			
Monday	Breakfast			
	Lunch			
	Dinner			
	Bedtime			
Tuesday	Breakfast			
	Lunch			
	Dinner			
	Bedtime			
Wednesday	Breakfast			
	Lunch			
	Dinner			
	Bedtime			
Thursday	Breakfast			
	Lunch			
	Dinner			
	Bedtime			
Friday	Breakfast			
	Lunch			
	Dinner			
	Bedtime			
Saturday	Breakfast			
	Lunch			
	Dinner			
	Bedtime			

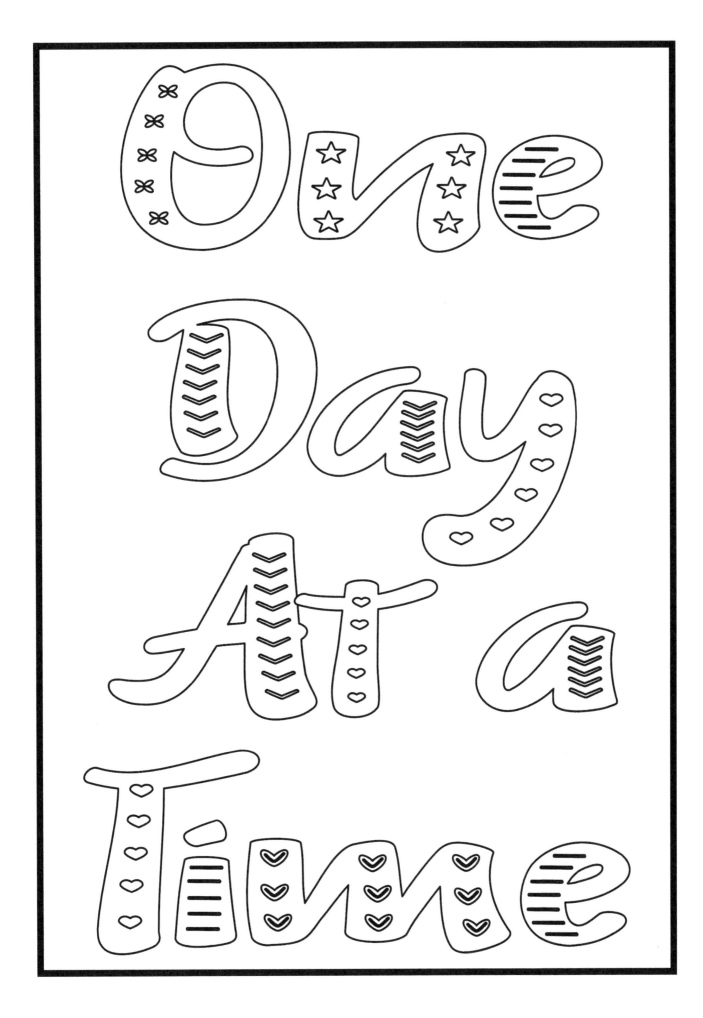

Blood Sugar Tracker

WEEK OF: _____

	Time	Before	After	Notes
Sunday	Breakfast			
	Lunch			
	Dinner			
	Bedtime			
Monday	Breakfast			
	Lunch			
	Dinner			
	Bedtime			
Tuesday	Breakfast			
	Lunch			
	Dinner			
	Bedtime			
Wednesday	Breakfast			
	Lunch			
	Dinner			
	Bedtime			
Thursday	Breakfast			
	Lunch			
	Dinner			
	Bedtime			
Friday	Breakfast			
	Lunch			
	Dinner			
	Bedtime			
Saturday	Breakfast			
	Lunch			
	Dinner			
	Bedtime			

Blood Sugar Tracker

WEEK OF: _____

Day	Time	Before	After	Notes
Sunday	Breakfast			
	Lunch			
	Dinner			
	Bedtime			
Monday	Breakfast			
	Lunch			
	Dinner			
	Bedtime			
Tuesday	Breakfast			
	Lunch			
	Dinner			
	Bedtime			
Wednesday	Breakfast			
	Lunch			
	Dinner			
	Bedtime			
Thursday	Breakfast			
	Lunch			
	Dinner			
	Bedtime			
Friday	Breakfast			
	Lunch			
	Dinner			
	Bedtime			
Saturday	Breakfast			
	Lunch			
	Dinner			
	Bedtime			

Blood Sugar Tracker

WEEK OF: _____

	Time	Before	After	Notes
Sunday	Breakfast			
	Lunch			
	Dinner			
	Bedtime			
Monday	Breakfast			
	Lunch			
	Dinner			
	Bedtime			
Tuesday	Breakfast			
	Lunch			
	Dinner			
	Bedtime			
Wednesday	Breakfast			
	Lunch			
	Dinner			
	Bedtime			
Thursday	Breakfast			
	Lunch			
	Dinner			
	Bedtime			
Friday	Breakfast			
	Lunch			
	Dinner			
	Bedtime			
Saturday	Breakfast			
	Lunch			
	Dinner			
	Bedtime			

Blood Sugar Tracker

WEEK OF: _____

Day	Time	Before	After	Notes
Sunday	Breakfast			
	Lunch			
	Dinner			
	Bedtime			
Monday	Breakfast			
	Lunch			
	Dinner			
	Bedtime			
Tuesday	Breakfast			
	Lunch			
	Dinner			
	Bedtime			
Wednesday	Breakfast			
	Lunch			
	Dinner			
	Bedtime			
Thursday	Breakfast			
	Lunch			
	Dinner			
	Bedtime			
Friday	Breakfast			
	Lunch			
	Dinner			
	Bedtime			
Saturday	Breakfast			
	Lunch			
	Dinner			
	Bedtime			

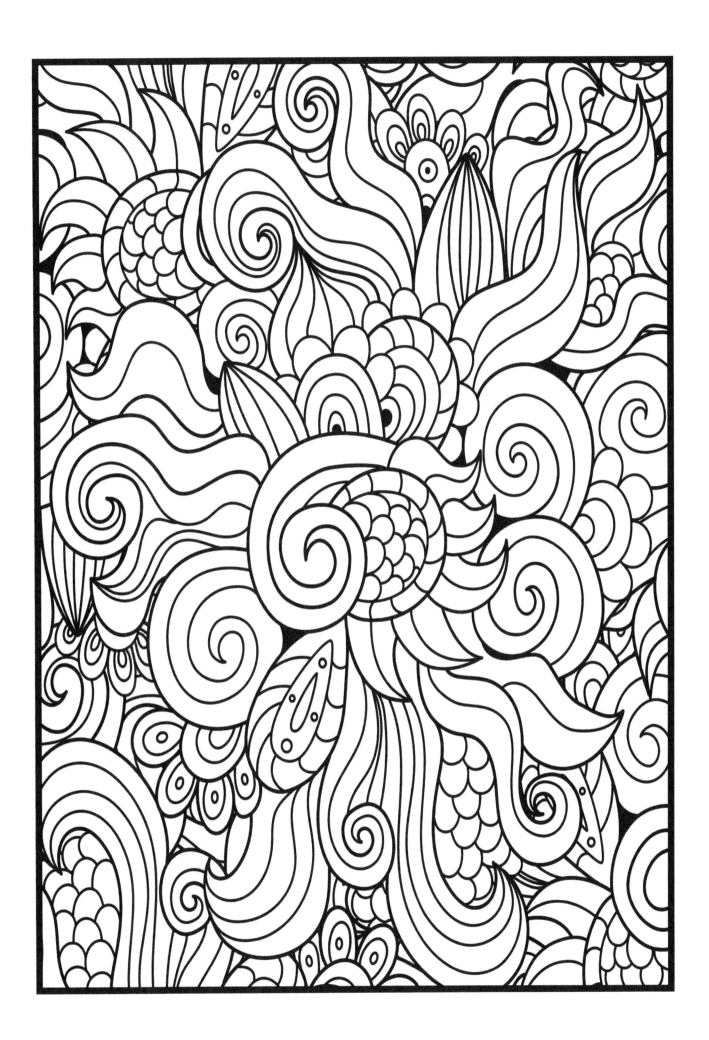

Blood Sugar Tracker

WEEK OF: _____

	Time	Before	After	Notes
Sunday	Breakfast			
	Lunch			
	Dinner			
	Bedtime			
Monday	Breakfast			
	Lunch			
	Dinner			
	Bedtime			
Tuesday	Breakfast			
	Lunch			
	Dinner			
	Bedtime			
Wednesday	Breakfast			
	Lunch			
	Dinner			
	Bedtime			
Thursday	Breakfast			
	Lunch			
	Dinner			
	Bedtime			
Friday	Breakfast			
	Lunch			
	Dinner			
	Bedtime			
Saturday	Breakfast			
	Lunch			
	Dinner			
	Bedtime			

Blood Sugar Tracker

WEEK OF: _____

	Time	Before	After	Notes
Sunday	Breakfast			
	Lunch			
	Dinner			
	Bedtime			
Monday	Breakfast			
	Lunch			
	Dinner			
	Bedtime			
Tuesday	Breakfast			
	Lunch			
	Dinner			
	Bedtime			
Wednesday	Breakfast			
	Lunch			
	Dinner			
	Bedtime			
Thursday	Breakfast			
	Lunch			
	Dinner			
	Bedtime			
Friday	Breakfast			
	Lunch			
	Dinner			
	Bedtime			
Saturday	Breakfast			
	Lunch			
	Dinner			
	Bedtime			

Blood Sugar Tracker

WEEK OF: _____

Day	Time	Before	After	Notes
Sunday	Breakfast			
	Lunch			
	Dinner			
	Bedtime			
Monday	Breakfast			
	Lunch			
	Dinner			
	Bedtime			
Tuesday	Breakfast			
	Lunch			
	Dinner			
	Bedtime			
Wednesday	Breakfast			
	Lunch			
	Dinner			
	Bedtime			
Thursday	Breakfast			
	Lunch			
	Dinner			
	Bedtime			
Friday	Breakfast			
	Lunch			
	Dinner			
	Bedtime			
Saturday	Breakfast			
	Lunch			
	Dinner			
	Bedtime			

Blood Sugar Tracker

WEEK OF: _____

	Time	Before	After	Notes
Sunday	Breakfast			
	Lunch			
	Dinner			
	Bedtime			
Monday	Breakfast			
	Lunch			
	Dinner			
	Bedtime			
Tuesday	Breakfast			
	Lunch			
	Dinner			
	Bedtime			
Wednesday	Breakfast			
	Lunch			
	Dinner			
	Bedtime			
Thursday	Breakfast			
	Lunch			
	Dinner			
	Bedtime			
Friday	Breakfast			
	Lunch			
	Dinner			
	Bedtime			
Saturday	Breakfast			
	Lunch			
	Dinner			
	Bedtime			

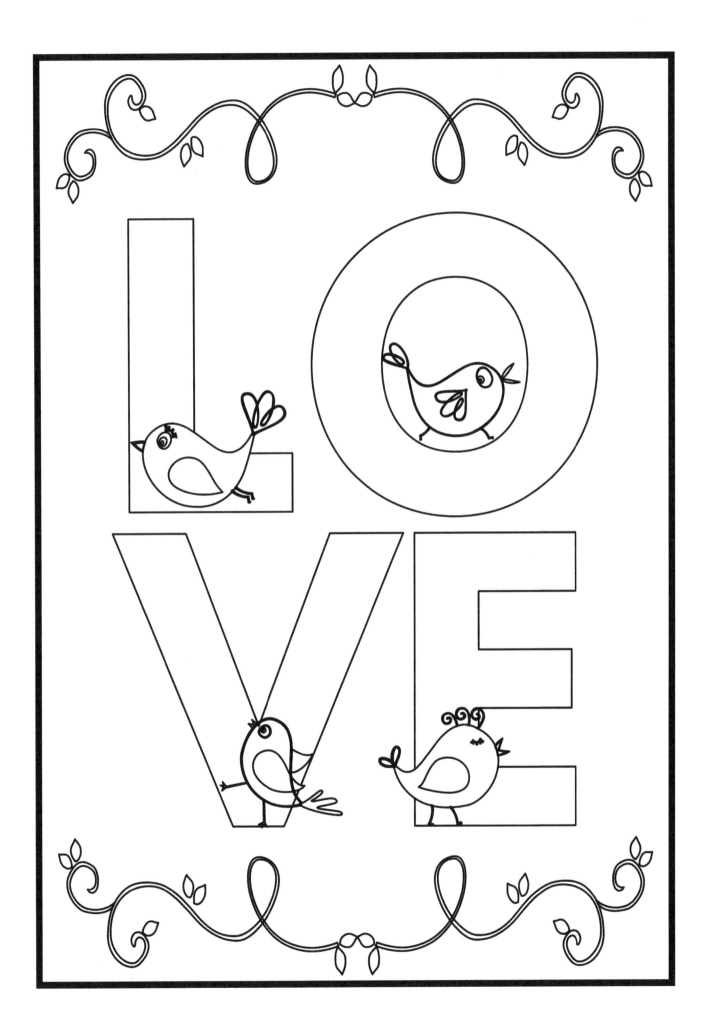

Blood Sugar Tracker

WEEK OF: _____

	Time	Before	After	Notes
Sunday	Breakfast			
	Lunch			
	Dinner			
	Bedtime			
Monday	Breakfast			
	Lunch			
	Dinner			
	Bedtime			
Tuesday	Breakfast			
	Lunch			
	Dinner			
	Bedtime			
Wednesday	Breakfast			
	Lunch			
	Dinner			
	Bedtime			
Thursday	Breakfast			
	Lunch			
	Dinner			
	Bedtime			
Friday	Breakfast			
	Lunch			
	Dinner			
	Bedtime			
Saturday	Breakfast			
	Lunch			
	Dinner			
	Bedtime			

Blood Sugar Tracker

WEEK OF: _____

	Time	Before	After	Notes
Sunday	Breakfast			
	Lunch			
	Dinner			
	Bedtime			
Monday	Breakfast			
	Lunch			
	Dinner			
	Bedtime			
Tuesday	Breakfast			
	Lunch			
	Dinner			
	Bedtime			
Wednesday	Breakfast			
	Lunch			
	Dinner			
	Bedtime			
Thursday	Breakfast			
	Lunch			
	Dinner			
	Bedtime			
Friday	Breakfast			
	Lunch			
	Dinner			
	Bedtime			
Saturday	Breakfast			
	Lunch			
	Dinner			
	Bedtime			

Blood Sugar Tracker

WEEK OF: _____

	Time	Before	After	Notes
Sunday	Breakfast			
	Lunch			
	Dinner			
	Bedtime			
Monday	Breakfast			
	Lunch			
	Dinner			
	Bedtime			
Tuesday	Breakfast			
	Lunch			
	Dinner			
	Bedtime			
Wednesday	Breakfast			
	Lunch			
	Dinner			
	Bedtime			
Thursday	Breakfast			
	Lunch			
	Dinner			
	Bedtime			
Friday	Breakfast			
	Lunch			
	Dinner			
	Bedtime			
Saturday	Breakfast			
	Lunch			
	Dinner			
	Bedtime			

Blood Sugar Tracker

WEEK OF: _____

	Time	Before	After	Notes
Sunday	Breakfast			
	Lunch			
	Dinner			
	Bedtime			
Monday	Breakfast			
	Lunch			
	Dinner			
	Bedtime			
Tuesday	Breakfast			
	Lunch			
	Dinner			
	Bedtime			
Wednesday	Breakfast			
	Lunch			
	Dinner			
	Bedtime			
Thursday	Breakfast			
	Lunch			
	Dinner			
	Bedtime			
Friday	Breakfast			
	Lunch			
	Dinner			
	Bedtime			
Saturday	Breakfast			
	Lunch			
	Dinner			
	Bedtime			

Blood Sugar Tracker

WEEK OF: _____

Day	Time	Before	After	Notes
Sunday	Breakfast			
	Lunch			
	Dinner			
	Bedtime			
Monday	Breakfast			
	Lunch			
	Dinner			
	Bedtime			
Tuesday	Breakfast			
	Lunch			
	Dinner			
	Bedtime			
Wednesday	Breakfast			
	Lunch			
	Dinner			
	Bedtime			
Thursday	Breakfast			
	Lunch			
	Dinner			
	Bedtime			
Friday	Breakfast			
	Lunch			
	Dinner			
	Bedtime			
Saturday	Breakfast			
	Lunch			
	Dinner			
	Bedtime			

Blood Sugar Tracker

WEEK OF: _____

Day	Time	Before	After	Notes
Sunday	Breakfast			
	Lunch			
	Dinner			
	Bedtime			
Monday	Breakfast			
	Lunch			
	Dinner			
	Bedtime			
Tuesday	Breakfast			
	Lunch			
	Dinner			
	Bedtime			
Wednesday	Breakfast			
	Lunch			
	Dinner			
	Bedtime			
Thursday	Breakfast			
	Lunch			
	Dinner			
	Bedtime			
Friday	Breakfast			
	Lunch			
	Dinner			
	Bedtime			
Saturday	Breakfast			
	Lunch			
	Dinner			
	Bedtime			

Blood Sugar Tracker

WEEK OF: _____

	Time	Before	After	Notes
Sunday	Breakfast			
	Lunch			
	Dinner			
	Bedtime			
Monday	Breakfast			
	Lunch			
	Dinner			
	Bedtime			
Tuesday	Breakfast			
	Lunch			
	Dinner			
	Bedtime			
Wednesday	Breakfast			
	Lunch			
	Dinner			
	Bedtime			
Thursday	Breakfast			
	Lunch			
	Dinner			
	Bedtime			
Friday	Breakfast			
	Lunch			
	Dinner			
	Bedtime			
Saturday	Breakfast			
	Lunch			
	Dinner			
	Bedtime			

Blood Sugar Tracker

WEEK OF: _____

Day	Time	Before	After	Notes
Sunday	Breakfast			
	Lunch			
	Dinner			
	Bedtime			
Monday	Breakfast			
	Lunch			
	Dinner			
	Bedtime			
Tuesday	Breakfast			
	Lunch			
	Dinner			
	Bedtime			
Wednesday	Breakfast			
	Lunch			
	Dinner			
	Bedtime			
Thursday	Breakfast			
	Lunch			
	Dinner			
	Bedtime			
Friday	Breakfast			
	Lunch			
	Dinner			
	Bedtime			
Saturday	Breakfast			
	Lunch			
	Dinner			
	Bedtime			

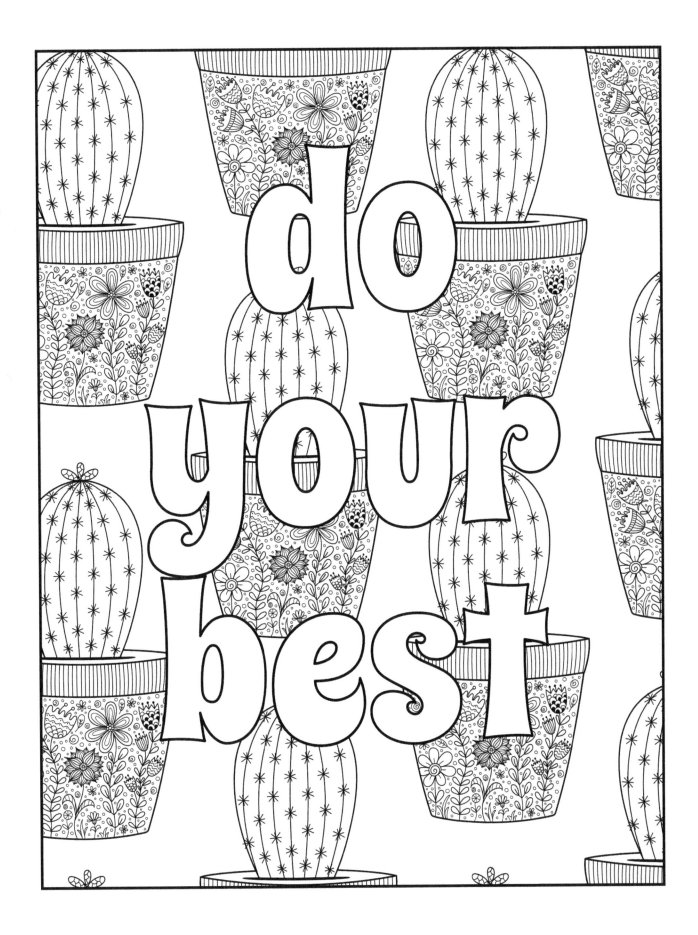

Blood Sugar Tracker

WEEK OF: _____

	Time	Before	After	Notes
Sunday	Breakfast			
	Lunch			
	Dinner			
	Bedtime			
Monday	Breakfast			
	Lunch			
	Dinner			
	Bedtime			
Tuesday	Breakfast			
	Lunch			
	Dinner			
	Bedtime			
Wednesday	Breakfast			
	Lunch			
	Dinner			
	Bedtime			
Thursday	Breakfast			
	Lunch			
	Dinner			
	Bedtime			
Friday	Breakfast			
	Lunch			
	Dinner			
	Bedtime			
Saturday	Breakfast			
	Lunch			
	Dinner			
	Bedtime			

Blood Sugar Tracker

WEEK OF: _____

	Time	Before	After	Notes
Sunday	Breakfast			
	Lunch			
	Dinner			
	Bedtime			
Monday	Breakfast			
	Lunch			
	Dinner			
	Bedtime			
Tuesday	Breakfast			
	Lunch			
	Dinner			
	Bedtime			
Wednesday	Breakfast			
	Lunch			
	Dinner			
	Bedtime			
Thursday	Breakfast			
	Lunch			
	Dinner			
	Bedtime			
Friday	Breakfast			
	Lunch			
	Dinner			
	Bedtime			
Saturday	Breakfast			
	Lunch			
	Dinner			
	Bedtime			

Blood Sugar Tracker

WEEK OF: _____

	Time	Before	After	Notes
Sunday	Breakfast			
	Lunch			
	Dinner			
	Bedtime			
Monday	Breakfast			
	Lunch			
	Dinner			
	Bedtime			
Tuesday	Breakfast			
	Lunch			
	Dinner			
	Bedtime			
Wednesday	Breakfast			
	Lunch			
	Dinner			
	Bedtime			
Thursday	Breakfast			
	Lunch			
	Dinner			
	Bedtime			
Friday	Breakfast			
	Lunch			
	Dinner			
	Bedtime			
Saturday	Breakfast			
	Lunch			
	Dinner			
	Bedtime			

Blood Sugar Tracker

WEEK OF: _____

	Time	Before	After	Notes
Sunday	Breakfast			
	Lunch			
	Dinner			
	Bedtime			
Monday	Breakfast			
	Lunch			
	Dinner			
	Bedtime			
Tuesday	Breakfast			
	Lunch			
	Dinner			
	Bedtime			
Wednesday	Breakfast			
	Lunch			
	Dinner			
	Bedtime			
Thursday	Breakfast			
	Lunch			
	Dinner			
	Bedtime			
Friday	Breakfast			
	Lunch			
	Dinner			
	Bedtime			
Saturday	Breakfast			
	Lunch			
	Dinner			
	Bedtime			

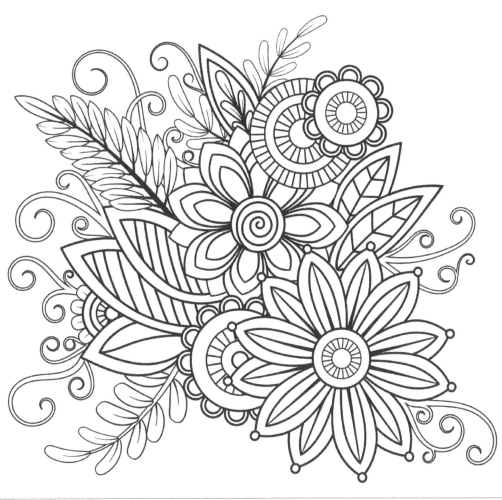

NOTES:

Blood Sugar Tracker

WEEK OF: _____

	Time	Before	After	Notes
Sunday	Breakfast			
	Lunch			
	Dinner			
	Bedtime			
Monday	Breakfast			
	Lunch			
	Dinner			
	Bedtime			
Tuesday	Breakfast			
	Lunch			
	Dinner			
	Bedtime			
Wednesday	Breakfast			
	Lunch			
	Dinner			
	Bedtime			
Thursday	Breakfast			
	Lunch			
	Dinner			
	Bedtime			
Friday	Breakfast			
	Lunch			
	Dinner			
	Bedtime			
Saturday	Breakfast			
	Lunch			
	Dinner			
	Bedtime			

Blood Sugar Tracker

WEEK OF: _____

	Time	Before	After	Notes
Sunday	Breakfast			
	Lunch			
	Dinner			
	Bedtime			
Monday	Breakfast			
	Lunch			
	Dinner			
	Bedtime			
Tuesday	Breakfast			
	Lunch			
	Dinner			
	Bedtime			
Wednesday	Breakfast			
	Lunch			
	Dinner			
	Bedtime			
Thursday	Breakfast			
	Lunch			
	Dinner			
	Bedtime			
Friday	Breakfast			
	Lunch			
	Dinner			
	Bedtime			
Saturday	Breakfast			
	Lunch			
	Dinner			
	Bedtime			

Blood Sugar Tracker

WEEK OF: _____

	Time	Before	After	Notes
Sunday	Breakfast			
	Lunch			
	Dinner			
	Bedtime			
Monday	Breakfast			
	Lunch			
	Dinner			
	Bedtime			
Tuesday	Breakfast			
	Lunch			
	Dinner			
	Bedtime			
Wednesday	Breakfast			
	Lunch			
	Dinner			
	Bedtime			
Thursday	Breakfast			
	Lunch			
	Dinner			
	Bedtime			
Friday	Breakfast			
	Lunch			
	Dinner			
	Bedtime			
Saturday	Breakfast			
	Lunch			
	Dinner			
	Bedtime			

Blood Sugar Tracker

WEEK OF: _____

	Time	Before	After	Notes
Sunday	Breakfast			
	Lunch			
	Dinner			
	Bedtime			
Monday	Breakfast			
	Lunch			
	Dinner			
	Bedtime			
Tuesday	Breakfast			
	Lunch			
	Dinner			
	Bedtime			
Wednesday	Breakfast			
	Lunch			
	Dinner			
	Bedtime			
Thursday	Breakfast			
	Lunch			
	Dinner			
	Bedtime			
Friday	Breakfast			
	Lunch			
	Dinner			
	Bedtime			
Saturday	Breakfast			
	Lunch			
	Dinner			
	Bedtime			

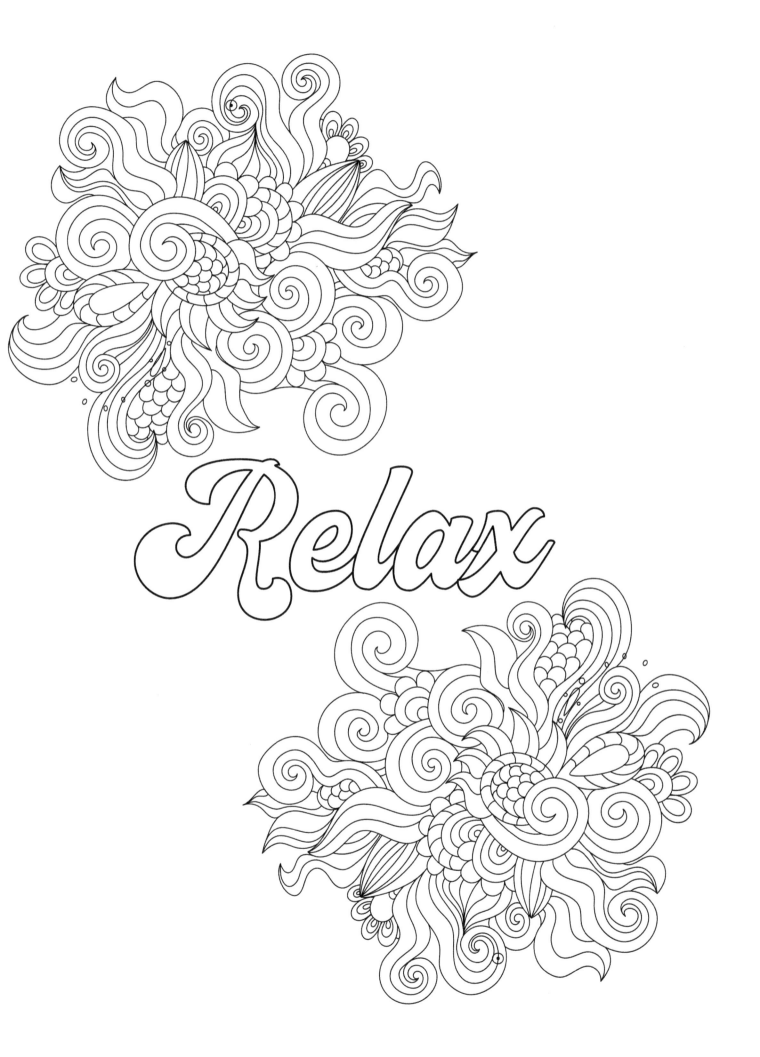

Blood Sugar Tracker

WEEK OF: _____

	Time	Before	After	Notes
Sunday	Breakfast			
	Lunch			
	Dinner			
	Bedtime			
Monday	Breakfast			
	Lunch			
	Dinner			
	Bedtime			
Tuesday	Breakfast			
	Lunch			
	Dinner			
	Bedtime			
Wednesday	Breakfast			
	Lunch			
	Dinner			
	Bedtime			
Thursday	Breakfast			
	Lunch			
	Dinner			
	Bedtime			
Friday	Breakfast			
	Lunch			
	Dinner			
	Bedtime			
Saturday	Breakfast			
	Lunch			
	Dinner			
	Bedtime			

Blood Sugar Tracker

WEEK OF: _____

	Time	Before	After	Notes
Sunday	Breakfast			
	Lunch			
	Dinner			
	Bedtime			
Monday	Breakfast			
	Lunch			
	Dinner			
	Bedtime			
Tuesday	Breakfast			
	Lunch			
	Dinner			
	Bedtime			
Wednesday	Breakfast			
	Lunch			
	Dinner			
	Bedtime			
Thursday	Breakfast			
	Lunch			
	Dinner			
	Bedtime			
Friday	Breakfast			
	Lunch			
	Dinner			
	Bedtime			
Saturday	Breakfast			
	Lunch			
	Dinner			
	Bedtime			

Blood Sugar Tracker

WEEK OF: _____

Day	Time	Before	After	Notes
Sunday	Breakfast			
	Lunch			
	Dinner			
	Bedtime			
Monday	Breakfast			
	Lunch			
	Dinner			
	Bedtime			
Tuesday	Breakfast			
	Lunch			
	Dinner			
	Bedtime			
Wednesday	Breakfast			
	Lunch			
	Dinner			
	Bedtime			
Thursday	Breakfast			
	Lunch			
	Dinner			
	Bedtime			
Friday	Breakfast			
	Lunch			
	Dinner			
	Bedtime			
Saturday	Breakfast			
	Lunch			
	Dinner			
	Bedtime			

Blood Sugar Tracker

WEEK OF: _____

Day	Time	Before	After	Notes
Sunday	Breakfast			
	Lunch			
	Dinner			
	Bedtime			
Monday	Breakfast			
	Lunch			
	Dinner			
	Bedtime			
Tuesday	Breakfast			
	Lunch			
	Dinner			
	Bedtime			
Wednesday	Breakfast			
	Lunch			
	Dinner			
	Bedtime			
Thursday	Breakfast			
	Lunch			
	Dinner			
	Bedtime			
Friday	Breakfast			
	Lunch			
	Dinner			
	Bedtime			
Saturday	Breakfast			
	Lunch			
	Dinner			
	Bedtime			

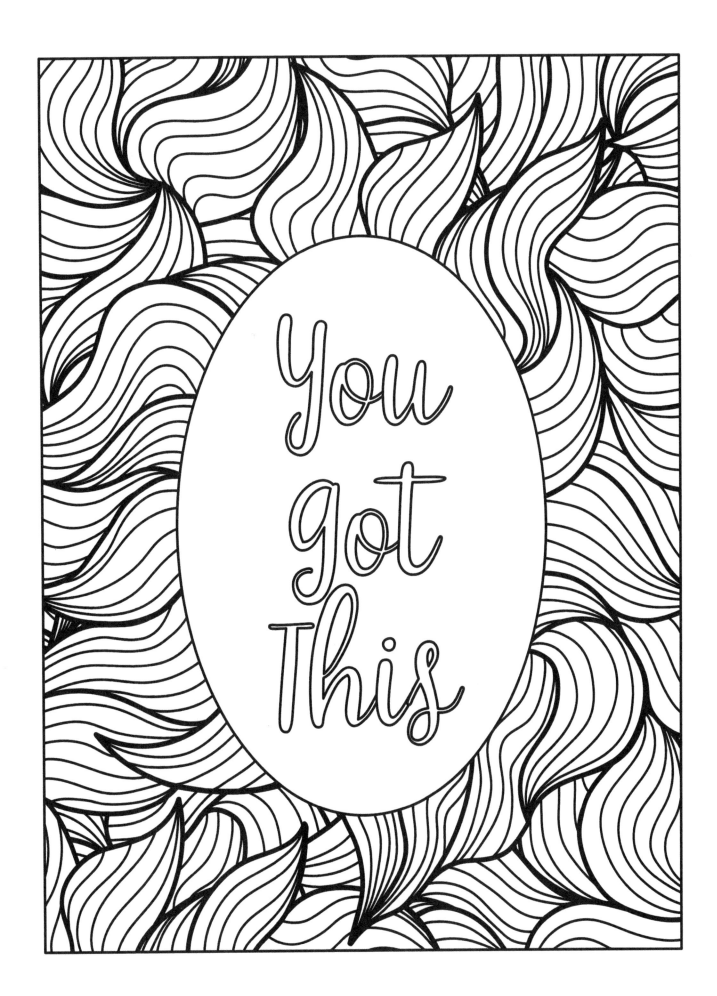

Blood Sugar Tracker

WEEK OF: _____

	Time	Before	After	Notes
Sunday	Breakfast			
	Lunch			
	Dinner			
	Bedtime			
Monday	Breakfast			
	Lunch			
	Dinner			
	Bedtime			
Tuesday	Breakfast			
	Lunch			
	Dinner			
	Bedtime			
Wednesday	Breakfast			
	Lunch			
	Dinner			
	Bedtime			
Thursday	Breakfast			
	Lunch			
	Dinner			
	Bedtime			
Friday	Breakfast			
	Lunch			
	Dinner			
	Bedtime			
Saturday	Breakfast			
	Lunch			
	Dinner			
	Bedtime			

Blood Sugar Tracker

WEEK OF: _____

Day	Time	Before	After	Notes
Sunday	Breakfast			
	Lunch			
	Dinner			
	Bedtime			
Monday	Breakfast			
	Lunch			
	Dinner			
	Bedtime			
Tuesday	Breakfast			
	Lunch			
	Dinner			
	Bedtime			
Wednesday	Breakfast			
	Lunch			
	Dinner			
	Bedtime			
Thursday	Breakfast			
	Lunch			
	Dinner			
	Bedtime			
Friday	Breakfast			
	Lunch			
	Dinner			
	Bedtime			
Saturday	Breakfast			
	Lunch			
	Dinner			
	Bedtime			

Blood Sugar Tracker

WEEK OF: _____

	Time	Before	After	Notes
Sunday	Breakfast			
	Lunch			
	Dinner			
	Bedtime			
Monday	Breakfast			
	Lunch			
	Dinner			
	Bedtime			
Tuesday	Breakfast			
	Lunch			
	Dinner			
	Bedtime			
Wednesday	Breakfast			
	Lunch			
	Dinner			
	Bedtime			
Thursday	Breakfast			
	Lunch			
	Dinner			
	Bedtime			
Friday	Breakfast			
	Lunch			
	Dinner			
	Bedtime			
Saturday	Breakfast			
	Lunch			
	Dinner			
	Bedtime			

Blood Sugar Tracker

WEEK OF: _____

	Time	Before	After	Notes
Sunday	Breakfast			
	Lunch			
	Dinner			
	Bedtime			
Monday	Breakfast			
	Lunch			
	Dinner			
	Bedtime			
Tuesday	Breakfast			
	Lunch			
	Dinner			
	Bedtime			
Wednesday	Breakfast			
	Lunch			
	Dinner			
	Bedtime			
Thursday	Breakfast			
	Lunch			
	Dinner			
	Bedtime			
Friday	Breakfast			
	Lunch			
	Dinner			
	Bedtime			
Saturday	Breakfast			
	Lunch			
	Dinner			
	Bedtime			

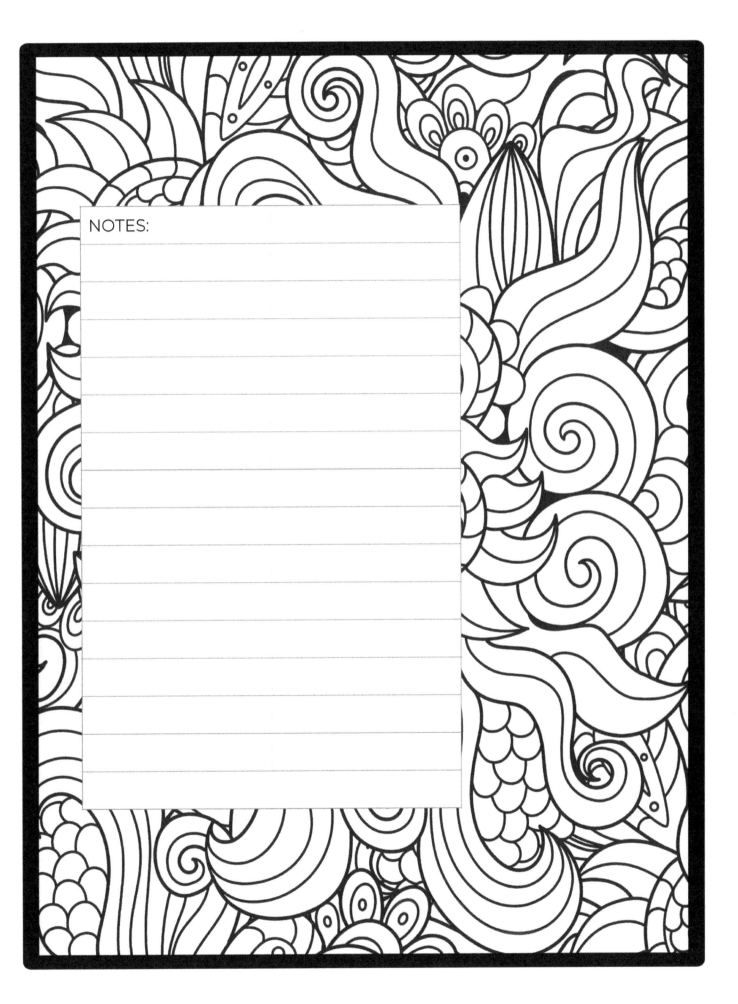

www.ingramcontent.com/pod-product-compliance
Lightning Source LLC
LaVergne TN
LVHW071103281224
800074LV00045B/2372